Directing your Life Script:

A Stress Management Workbook

Dr. Gina Pazzaglia

DEDICATION

This workbook is dedicated to those who have suffered from experiences
that have negatively impacted their life script.

CONTENTS

This workbook is a guide for helping you imagine what you would like your life to look like. You will be able to better understand how stress has impacted your view of life and healthier ways to deal with stress. As you go through these pages, you will learn to re-write your *life script*. As you write it, you will discover that you can manage the stress you feel so that **you** control it.
It will no longer control you.
This is a workbook with practical strategies and practice sections.

ACKNOWLEDGMENTS

I would like to acknowledge those who have helped me throughout a lifetime.
Those who have challenged me with strategies to manage and change
my own life script.
This includes gratitude to my God, many professors,
educators as well as a vast variety of life's trials,
that inevitably have facilitated my growth
in teaching stress management strategies.

1 OUR LIFE SCRIPT

First of all, think about your life as a movie, how do you like the movie so far? If you don't like it, or think it needs improving, guess what? You are the director and writer of your *life script.* Your current *life script* has already been written, based on many different factors, and it has been imprinted in your subconscious mind.

To achieve the life you were **meant to live**; your goal, as the director of your movie, must be to uncover the script in your *subconscious mind*, and to learn to observe your script with objectivity. You must try to learn to embrace what has happened in your life, in your script, thus far. Then you may be able to decide, as the director and writer of your own *life script,* to change the dynamics, and the actors. Thus, you can re-write your script, when necessary.

Now that you understand a little about the *life script* that has been written in your subconscious mind, try this exercise so that it will become even clearer.

Exercise

Breathe deeply, taking air in through your nose, then letting it out through your mouth.

Breathe in, pushing your diaphragm (stomach) out, then exhale out more air than you took in, retracting your stomach.

Imagine yourself sitting in a director's chair,

just like a movie director. Imagine that a

movie begins to play,

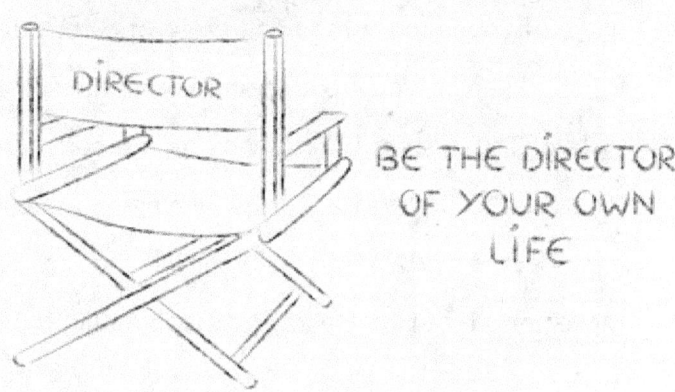

and it is all about your life.

Continue your breathing as you open your heart to love, and you open your heart to a greater sense of wholeness. Allow loving feelings to flow toward you.

Now, imagine yourself as a child and allow love to flow toward you as a child.

Give your *child-self* your loving guidance, and a desire to achieve a greater sense of wholeness.

Continue your breathing. Stay with the scene in front of you, the scene of your

child-self, with love and guidance and a sense of wholeness.

❖Can you see yourself as a child? See yourself as a carefree, playful, creative child, unencumbered by life problems.

❖If so, you can see how your subconscious mind wants you to live life, fully and freely.

❖If not, perhaps you have had a troubled life, with traumatic events that are keeping some areas of your brain from allowing you to access your child-self, your real self. Your child-self is full of faith, creativity, and curiosity; your child-self is carefree, hopeful, full of love, kindness, generosity, and many other of the attributes of children before they encounter life's troubles, trials, misfortunes, and traumatic events.

❖If you saw images that brought you discomfort, and your mind preferred to block these memories, you may want to practice the above exercise again. As you continue your breathing, and imagine yourself in your director's chair, and see your child-self with love, guidance, and a sense of wholeness, try to remember a time when you were happy and felt safe and secure.

❖❖For those of you with Posttraumatic Stress Disorder (PTSD) related to your childhood, and those of you who cannot bring times of carefree happiness to your imagination, do not worry. What's keeping you from seeing your child-self in its original state is a very strong defense system. This system is like a box of memories your child-self, and your older, emotional-self, feels are too harmful or overwhelming to remember. Unfortunately, this system of your mind has selected certain times of your life that are too traumatic, and it has blocked memories of those periods of your life, rather than treating them one memory at a time. This system of your mind, when you have been exposed to a traumatic event or situation, is called the **memory-consolidator**, and it is very protective. Even so, sometimes you must prove to yourself that you can handle and know how to manage uncomfortable, traumatic memories.

As you work through this workbook, you will be taking some very strong, powerful steps, and your emotional-self will begin to trust your mind to release more memories.

❖❖ This blocking of your memories, or your exposure to a traumatic event in your childhood, may indicate you would benefit further from the help of a therapist, since, sometimes, bad memories that happened for too long, were too painful, or were too frightening, caused PTSD symptoms, such as panic attacks; night terrors; erratic moods; feelings of distrust; insomnia; and other problems. Those symptoms arise from your feeling helpless ad vulnerable because you could not fight or run away, so the memory of those traumatic events is inside you and causes your body to react. You may feel pressure in your chest, or have heart palpitations, or shortness of breath. If those things happen too often, they can cause your brain pathways to malfunction, or to short-circuit. In that case, you may need more intense energy work, such as Qi Gong, Thought Field Therapy, EMDR, hypnotherapy, medications, essential oil therapy, or other adjunct services or products, besides therapy.

❖❖If you are able to continue here, follow the next set of instructions; if not, you may wish to stop and consult a therapist who will help you with your PTSD symptoms.

Now that you have observed the scene of your *child-self* in its original, free, happy, creative state, write about that scene, as yourself, the director of it. If you prefer, draw what you saw.

Write about the scene you saw as the director and the impressions about it

_____

_____

_____

_____

_____

_____

_____

_____

If you felt or saw images that brought you discomfort, and your mind prefers to block good memories, then you may want to practice the above exercise again. Specifically attempt to remember a time when you were happy and felt safe and secure. BREATHE DEEPLY, TAKING AIR IN THROUGH YOUR NOSE, THEN LETTING IT OUTH THROUGH YOUR MOUTH. BREATHE IN, AND THEN BREATHE OUT EVEN MORE AIR THAN YOU INHALED.

WRITE OR DRAW THE NEW SCENE:

_____

_____

_____   _____

See, your mind is both able and willing to imagine. This means it is also able to visualize new scenes. Scenes of what you want and desire in your life. Sometimes, it is *stress* that inhibits us from being able to imagine and hope for more benefits in our lives.

Understanding stress in very important towards writing and re-writing our scripts in life.

2 What is Stress?

Stress can be defined as the response of the human organism to any change or demand. Whether the demand or stress is positive or negative, the body responds automatically. Stress has three parts: It is perceptual, physical, and emotional. Stress is **perceptual** because it has to do with the way you see and understand things; it's like a lens you are looking through to make sense of what is happening in your life. Stress is **physical** because it is a set of sensations and symptoms that you experience in your body. Stress is **emotional**, because it includes a set of feelings you may have, like anxiety, fear, or helplessness.

How Can I Understand Stress?

To understand stress you need to identify what stress causes you to think and believe (perception); what it causes your body to experience (physical); and what it causes you to feel (emotion).

So Let's Start With Stress as a Set of Perceptions:

Imagine that you were originally created and designed to enjoy life; to have success; and to have positive relationships.

That's wonderful, isn't it?

That's what most people want for themselves.

If those are aspects of your life that you want, and that you find pleasurable, why do so many people seldom feel that pleasure, that enjoyment?

What Stress Can and Cannot Do Is Up To You

There are many things in life that can cause suffering, but does that mean you cannot live the life for which you were designed? Of course not. You can find pleasure and enjoyment, even when stressful events and situations occur.

Perceiving an event or situation as stress-free, or stress-ful occurs in your subconscious mind. Your **subconscious mind** is really not the murky and mysterious place you may have thought it was. Your subconscious mind is where you can find the magic of recovering what is rightfully yours --your wonderfully fulfilled, enjoyable and pleasurable life.

Yes, you have suffered. You have had, and maybe will have pain, loss, and things you cannot control.

Despite the negative and painful things in your life, it is deep inside your subconscious mind where you have the ability to transform yourself and your life. Your subconscious mind is where you become what you were meant to be on this earth, and in your body.

You can take your bad experiences and put them in the *life script* of your story, so that you can refine, help, and restore your positive virtues and character.

Ultimately, this may make you see yourself as happy, fulfilled, loving, creative, and enduring, no matter what the circumstances were, or what the circumstances may be.

That sounds wonderful, but you want to know how that can be true, and what you need to do to make it come true.

Understanding Past, Present and Future

When we see our past, it is often latent with regrets that impact our emotional mood maybe stimulating feelings of despair, helplessness and fear. If we understand regret as we look upon events and situations we could not control, or that ended up badly, we can turn regrets into opportunities.

We can only activate the change process in the Present, or as many refer to as "the Now." At this point of the present, we can emotionally review our history from a perspective of opportunity, and change the meaning of the event. Thus, this creates immediate change in the future because we will respond and interact in our world in a different way-Re-writing our life script.

So let's go a little deeper and realize how to begin this process. First, we must understand **Stress** and all the perspectives of stress (perceptual, physical, and emotional).

In this workbook, reflect on your life as objectively as you can, as your own director of your life.

Try to determine the changes you need to make so you can see, feel, think about, observe and then use to improve your life script.

You can determine what changes you need to make, and want to make, so you can recreate some of those wonderful characteristics of your free, happy child-self to make your adult-self feel less like you are a victim and more like you are an overcomer!

It is your life; make it the best story ever!

Beliefs are the underlying **boxes** in your subconscious mind. The **subconscious mind** is the place where you construct **meaning formation.** Meaning formation is how you make **sense** and **safety** in the world around you. The **problem** is, **meaning formation** is often **restrictive** and **inflexible.** To overcome those obstacles to your meaning-making, you need to **"think outside the box"**

Belief boxes create **mental filters** and **defenses** to try to keep us safe and secure, often **from** things that are **past** memories or experiences.

Beliefs →feelings→ thoughts → are the triggers to the **CNS** (central nervous system) response **(Fight, Flight, Freeze or Friendly)**

Perceptual Stress:

What makes one person feel stressed may have no effect on another person. Your perceptions, the way you relate to stress, and how you structure your beliefs are what determine the sense of empowerment or dis-empowerment you feel in the world around you, and how you relate to stress. Stress will often hit your fight, flight, fear, freeze and friendly reactive systems.

If you find yourself looking through mud colored glasses, rather than rose colored glasses, don't worry….That can change!!!

Stress is based on personal experience:

Has anything recently happened that has made you feel overwhelmed?

_____

_____

_____ _____

Does what happened remind you of a bad experience from my past? If so, what?

_____

_____

_____ _____

Stress is based on personality and family personality styles

There are some personality traits that get passed down through family systems and how they perceive and react to stressful events, beliefs, and experiences. Below are some examples. You have a space to talk about the traits passed down as normal in your family.

Do you have a personality that tends to get overly anxious, worried or fearful? A family may believe if you're not worried, you don't care. Or, that it is irresponsible if you do not worry.

_____

_____

_____ _____

Were you taught to believe it is normal to be irritable and anxious about anything that is out of your control?

_____

_____

_____ _____

Another common family personality trait is to take care of everyone but yourself. Do you believe to take care of yourself means you are selfish?

_____

_____

_____ _____

Does your family eat when upset or are they inactive (couch potatoes)?

_____

_____

_____ _____

Does your family gossip and are they vindictive?

_____

_____

_____ _____

Does your family try to please everyone?

_____

_____

_____

 Does your family expect perfection?

_____

_____

_____

Does your family system use guilt as a motivator?

_____

_____

_____

Does your family believe criticism helps make you better?

_____

_____

_____

Does your family refuse to ask for help because that is considered a weakness?

_____

_____

_____

Does your family use anger or silence as a means to control one another?

_____

_____

_____

Do any of those examples fit you? I hope you took the time to write a little after those that apply. That is how you know some about your current life script.

Are there other traits you remember from your family?

_____

_____

_____

Stress is based on self-view

Ask yourself:

Am I critical of myself? How:

_____

_____

_____

Do I expect myself to be perfect?

_____

_____

_____

What is unrealistic about my expectations of myself?

_____

_____

_____

Did my family teach me to think too highly of myself, if so what negative outcomes have happened as a result? (such as people think I am stuck up; people say I am arrogant, etc).

_____

_____

_____

Do I have an exaggerated sense of self-importance to cover the shame I feel about who I really am? If so, what shame issues have happened to me?

_____

_____

_____

Do I believe I was a mistake? Talk about feeling like a mistake.

_____

_____

_____

Do I believe I am worthless? What triggers make you feel worthless? Talk about it.

_____

_____

_____

I hope you took the time to write about these that apply.

Are there other self-views you have that have negatively impacted you?

_____

_____

What are some of the negative or critical things you tell yourself in relationship to others? For example, I say negative things about myself... *when I try to speak to my boss* (peer, in-laws, etc.)

I say negative things when I _____

I say negative things when I _____

I say negative things when I _____

Now, list the critical things you tell yourself. For example, I will never be as good as my sister (friend, co-worker, brother, spouse)

I say critical things such as: I _____

I say critical things such as: I _____

I say critical things such as: I _____

Stress is based on culture and environmental expectations.

Ask yourself if others outside of yourself expect you to take care of things that are really not your responsibility. Such as your work, church, school, cultural beliefs and practices, as well as ethnicity. An example is when you work full time, but your church expects you to attend and volunteer at every service. If so, who and/or what are they? Describe what they expect of you.

_____

_____

_____

Physical Stress Includes:

- The rate of wear and tear on your body
- Your body's reactions to physical, chemical, or emotional changes
- Your body's reactions to environmental changes (e.g., new surroundings)
- Your body's response to things that threaten, scare, worry, or excite you.

Examples of Physical Stress:

- Injury

- Illness

- Extreme temperature changes

- Exhaustion

- Elation

- Sitting or standing still too long

- Moving too fast, or for too long

- Working at a task too long

Learning to recognize early **physical signs of stress** can assist you in managing it. Asking yourself questions like:

Is my stomach hurting (or my head, my muscles)? How long has it been hurting?

Am I having unusual aches and pains in my joints?

Am I having unusual aches and pains elsewhere in my body? Do I have nervous energy?

Am I clenching my fists? Has my respiration changed? Am I holding my breath?

What are your symptoms?

_____

_____

_____

These are all signs your body is giving you that indicate you are having a stress reaction and you need to consider:

What are any recent changes or events that may be contributing to your stress levels? (Examples- travel, risk taking behaviors, recent illness, poor sleep, eating junk food, etc.)

_____

_____

_____

Am I doing too much? If yes, what can I cut out?

_____

_____

_____

Am I getting enough rest? If not, why?

_____

_____

_____

What are ways I have attempted, but have not worked?

_____

_____

_____

What are some ways I can improve my rest?

_____

_____

_____

Stress is Emotional

Types of Emotional Stress

Fear

Fear is a response to change and to the unknown.

Do you find yourself being fearful of things that might happen? If so, what are those fears and how do they relate to your past?

_____

_____

_____

Ask yourself:

What things do I see around me that make me feel afraid?

_____

_____

_____

What situations do I feel I should be able to control, but can't?

_____

_____

_____

What things have happened to me in the past that I am afraid will happen again?

_____

_____

_____

What makes me fearful about the future?

_____

_____

_____

Do you find yourself being afraid of your environment, where you live, who you live with, your office, school, neighborhood, etc.? If so, who, where, or what makes you feel afraid?

_____

_____

_____

Are you afraid you may lose someone close to you, if so, who and why?

_____

_____

_____

Are you afraid of being rejected, abandoned or hurt emotionally? If, so who and what makes you feel like that?

_____

_____

_____

Is that feeling of fear of rejection or abandonment, or emotional pain related to past hurts?

_____

_____

_____

Are you sure it is a real fear? How can you tell?

_____

_____

_____

If it isn't real fear, what could you tell yourself differently?

_____

_____

_____

How does fear keep you from changing?

_____

_____

_____

What situations would be better if you didn't resist the change?

_____

_____

_____

What changes have happened despite your resistance?

_____

_____

_____

3 Is Stress Good or Bad?

We are all under stress daily. Without it, we wouldn't move, think, get out of bed, or even care.

Humans thrive on stress. *It is a motivator.*

Body Responses

Although your mind distinguishes between good and bad stress, your body doesn't. Stress produces energy that can be beneficial or detrimental. For instance, you get a promotion and it brings stress to perform better, but it also brings excitement about the related increase in your pay. Both stresses are energy; both can be positive energy if directed correctly, both can be negative energy if invoked by fear.

You can be afraid you won't perform correctly, thus creating anxious feelings perceptually, emotionally, and physically. Perhaps you were told you would never amount to anything, or you were told everything you did was wrong or messed up. If either were the case, you may become anxious about getting a promotion and you may feel new pressure.

On the other hand, if you grew up believing in yourself and being confident, then a promotion and the positive stress about it could produce good **dopamine** (a brain chemical that enhances a feeling of well-being) towards goal setting and creative thinking, all resulting in good energy.

Your stress is managed differently by the energy you produce.

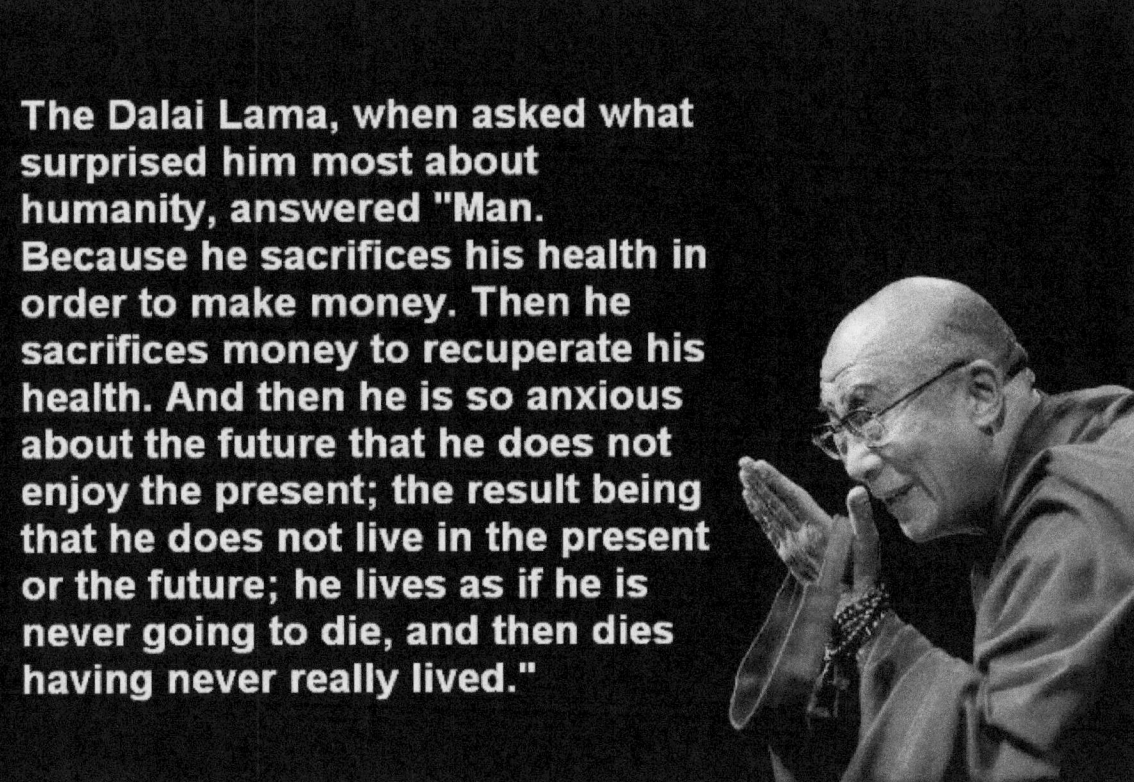

The Dalai Lama, when asked what surprised him most about humanity, answered "Man. Because he sacrifices his health in order to make money. Then he sacrifices money to recuperate his health. And then he is so anxious about the future that he does not enjoy the present; the result being that he does not live in the present or the future; he lives as if he is never going to die, and then dies having never really lived."

What energy drives you? Is it fearful energy?

Is it the energy from excitement?

What physical sensations of energy do you get when you are afraid?

_____

_____

How does negative, fearful energy affect your goals and drives?

_____

_____

_____

What sensations do you get when you are enthusiastic and excited?

_____

_____

_____

What does that positive energy motivate you to do?

_____

_____

_____

Does that energy affect you badly? If so, how?

_____

_____

_____

Action

Stress that produces positive energy prompts us to do certain things, at times.

What do you usually do when you are enthusiastic or confident? What things do you do when your energy is positive?

_____

_____

_____

What actions benefit you when you are enthusiastic or confident? (example: I am more likely to follow through with a goal).

_____

_____

_____

What are actions you can do to increase your enthusiastic, confident energy?

_____

_____

_____

Stress and Diet

The body's response to stress can directly and indirectly affect your nutritional states; stress can affect your appetite, the amount you eat, and the kinds of foods you eat. Ask yourself:

Am I eating properly and regularly?

Has my appetite increased? Has my appetite decreased?

Have I changed what I am eating?

Am I eating or drinking things that are bad for me (caffeine, alcohol, sugar, salt, fats, and artificial additives)?

Put a check mark by each example that applies to you.

What other signs are there that your body's nutritional state has changed?

_____

_____

_____

_____

_____

_____

What are some ways you can improve your nutrition?

_____

_____

_____

_____

_____

_____

Long-term Physical Factors

*Age, * Sex, *Genetics, *Chronic Disease, etc.

Stress is affected by, and affects you, depending on your age, sex, genetics, and state of health. For example, as you age, your metabolism may change, so you may eat the same amount you did when you were younger, but your body does not process what you eat as quickly and efficiently.

Are your expectations of yourself reasonable for your age, genetics, gender, and physical circumstances? An example could be: You are 65 years old; you are still in a full-time career; you have chronic pain from surgery; and you are caring for an aging parent. Too much...

Based on your own characteristics, what is realistic and reasonable, in terms of your expectations of yourself?

_____

_____

_____

Based on your own characteristics, what are the realistic, reasonable factors that help you decide when you need help?

_____

_____

_____

Stress is Psychological

Predictability

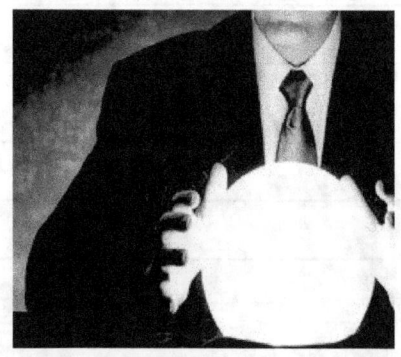

Predictability tends to assist us in decreasing anxiety. However, it can also diminish appropriate risks that may offer great opportunities to build new chemical pathways related to success, experience, goals, etc.

Ask yourself:

In my life, what is predictable and helps me deal with anxiety or depression?

_____

_____

_____

In my life, what is monotonous and makes me more fearful of making changes or taking risks?

_____

_____

_____

Frustration outlets

Having some defined frustration outlets, and creating some new ones, can help you deal with stress. For example, some people take out their stress-related frustrations through intense, physical exercise. Ask yourself:

What are my frustration outlets? If I don't have any, what can my frustration outlets be?

_____

_____

_____

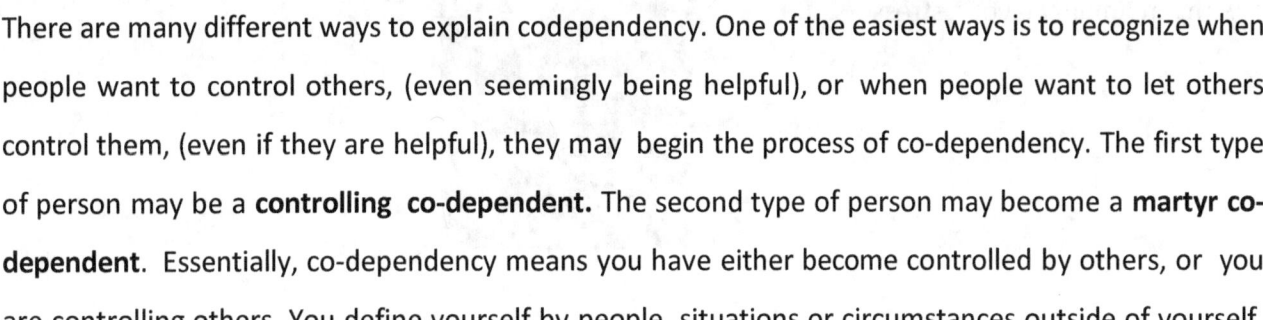

Stress and codependency

What is codependency?

There are many different ways to explain codependency. One of the easiest ways is to recognize when people want to control others, (even seemingly being helpful), or when people want to let others control them, (even if they are helpful), they may begin the process of co-dependency. The first type of person may be a **controlling co-dependent.** The second type of person may become a **martyr co-dependent**. Essentially, co-dependency means you have either become controlled by others, or you are controlling others. You define yourself by people, situations or circumstances outside of yourself. You have lost your own autonomy (individuality).

Do you feel you need to control what happens to others (e.g., how your teenager dresses; what your spouse does recreationally; how a family member engages with others in the family)? How do you need to control what happens to others?

_____

_____

_____

Do you feel you need to be controlled by others (e.g., being told by your spouse what you can spend; being told where you can and cannot go, and whom you can and cannot see)? How do you need to be controlled by others?

_____

_____

_____

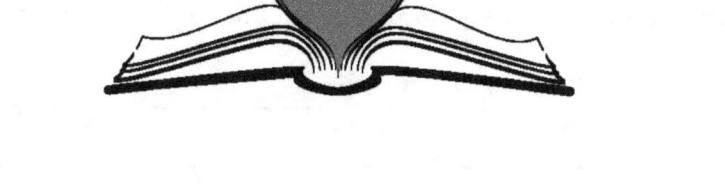

Now, you may realize there are things you would like to rewrite in your *life script*. If you have honestly answered these questions, and worked through the sections of this workbook, you are ready to re-write your script. By answering these questions you have identified your stress, and are learning how you deal with, and manage your stressors.

4 LIVING NEW

Now the fun part begins!

Now is when you learn to practice the process, like a new actor practices a fresh script. The words and actions in an old script come easily, but now you can rewrite it!

Below are some quick reminders of immediate *life script* inserts that will help you. Practice is going to make you proud as the director of your life!

Practice the first breathing exercise and imagine yourself now and/or in the future. Place yourself in a safe and familiar location in your visual image. Now, you can insert the affirmations below. Take at least one or two affirmations a day that are relevant to how you want to write your story. Imagine yourself feeling them, and what you would look like and feel, if you have these qualities.

Affirmations:

When speaking these affirmations to yourself, get in a relaxed state, and allow yourself to generate each feeling and image about yourself.

I love myself

I take good care of myself

I love and accept my body

I am good to my body and my body is good to me

I love my body, it carries my spirit around

I deserve to be happy

I forgive those who have hurt me

I love deeply

I deserve to be full of energy and vitality

I deserve to be healthy and feel good about myself

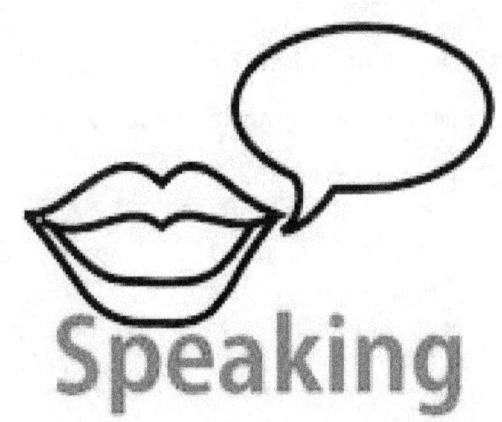

I am naturally attractive just the way I am

I am growing to be more attractive each day

I am warm and compassionate

I am creative

I have strength of character

I am wise in my judgment

I have serenity

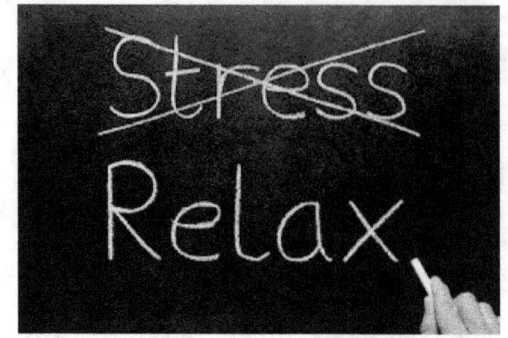

Stress Reduction Affirmations

1. Make your Life Dream board

I remember my first dream board. It was before I had lost weight and before I had entered a PhD program. I cut out a beautiful body and put my head on it. I cut out a diploma and cut out the letters **P h D**. I glued these on a board and put it on my refrigerator. Within 6 months, I had lost 10 pounds and had begun my PhD program. Within 2 years, I had lost the weight I wanted to lose and several years later, completed my PhD.

- A dream board can be a variety of things: you can take a poster board, and find pictures of how you want to see yourself (using letters, objects, phrases, etc).

- You can find pictures on the internet or you can cut up magazines.

- You can make it a collage (overlapping and non structured, or you can make it structured...)

- Be creative!

2. Make a Mind movie-a small video reflecting what you want in your life. You can use a program from mindmovie.com

3. Use your imagination with emotion and feeling for what you want or goals you have.

- It is important to gather as many sensory feelings as you can during the imagination. Such as the smell, the taste, the temperature, the time of day, the sounds around you, the lighting, the location, where you are sitting or what you are doing.

Two years ago, I wanted to do more traveling, so at night, I began to see myself, in great detail (What I had on, the temperature outside, getting on a plane or driving, arriving at the destination and feeling excited, etc). Over the last two years, I have made several amazing trips that were very similar to the imaginations I had created months and years before.

4. Balance your work and recreation

5. Exercise doing cardio if possible

6. Make sure you have a proper nutrition

7. Talk it out

8. Accept your limitations, and the limitations of others

9. Determine your responsibility

10. Determine your boundaries

11. Get enough rest

12. Work off stress and frustration with positive activities

13. Use Energy Healing Strategies such as Yoga and Qi Gong

I hope this workbook has been beneficial and you are beginning to see yourself in a new Life Script. If you have had trouble with these activities, it may benefit you to seek professional counseling to you get past some of your stuck places.

You can find further workbooks by visiting our website restorativealternativewellness.org

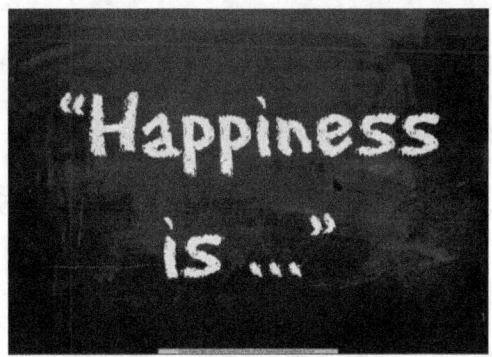

ABOUT THE AUTHOR

Gina Pazzaglia is a published author of the Trilogy: Celestine Algorithms, and owner of Restorative Alternative Wellness, LLC. She completed her Bachelor's degree in social work from Oral Roberts University, Master's degree in social work from University of Oklahoma, PhD abd from North Central University, and her PhD from the Graduate Theological Foundation, Mishawaka, Indiana. She is a Licensed Clinical Social Worker, Licensed Drug and Alcohol counselor, a state board certified supervisor for LCSW and LADC, she has been an ordained elder for several local churches, and a certified domestic violence counselor. She was founder and director of a not for profit mental health agency for almost ten years, and has over 20 years of experience treating persons suffering from emotional, physical and spiritual injuries.

Gina has had the opportunity to be a featured speaker at workshops and conferences, radio talk shows and television networks discussing various mental health and relationship topics, as well as offering leadership guidance for a variety of organizations. Gina is former co-owner of the Beatnix Café, Inc. She is a mother of five children, six grandchildren (and multiplying), and has dealt with many personal losses in her life to provide ample life enhancing experiences.

Gina has provided individual, family and group counseling in multiple specialty areas, especially related to abuse and trauma. She is dedicated to continue to bring positive and restorative help to those who have endured pain and heartache from mental, emotional, physical, relational, and spiritual losses.